MW01147717

To my parents,

Thank you for your love, support and guidance.

To my clients,

Thank you for the inspiration, motivation,
and so many pertinent life lessons.

John Monteleone

About This Book

This book is written in two main sections.

In Part 1, we'll explore the concept of retirement and what a successful retirement looks like from the angle of health and fitness. Then, since history is my biggest passion after fitness, we'll have a look at the history of exercise and how and why our collective activity level took a nosedive during the 20th century.

We'll also examine five myths of aging, and why they are just that – myths. Then we'll finish Part 1 with a wrap up of why exercise is so important, not only physically, but mentally and emotionally, as well. Many studies indicate that physical activity reduces depression and anxiety, while enhancing self-esteem and confidence.

Part 2 reads a little more like an instruction manual, in that it covers the logistics of getting started in an exercise routine, goal setting, establishing a routine and so forth. You'll also read descriptions and see photos of exercises that would be beneficial to incorporate in your routine.

And, we'll end with a chapter on what to be aware of when you're looking for a gym and a personal trainer. Interspersed throughout the book you'll find some additional information intended to motivate and inform you.

I have a lot of great clients, but there are some who

are particularly inspiring. I've shared some of their stories in extended sidebars. There are several other types of sidebars, as well, offering fitness tips, reliable sites for additional information and just some interesting snippets of information.

Finally, the book begins and ends with recaps of two Sunday morning phone calls with my father, also John Monteleone. Many of my Sundays begin with a phone call from my dad. It's always the best part of my day, and I thought I'd share a couple of them with you.

A Sunday Conversation with My Dad

It's 6 a.m. on a Sunday and the phone rings.

"Hi Dad! How are you doing?"

My father, 30 years retired Army who has been 10 years out of uniform, replies: "I'm good son. Not much going on here; I wanted to call to see how you are doing. I'm getting ready for the planting season."

In my opinion, my father was born in the wrong century. His idea about "getting back to the basics" is something that has permeated his personal philosophy as long as I can remember and is evidenced by our early morning talks. No need to burn sunlight when we can speak at 6 a.m., right?

Not one to rest on his laurels after his long military service, and frankly, he probably was just bored, Dad opened his own gunsmith shop, handcrafting flintlock rifles.

After 10 years of successfully running that business, he again got restless and decided to close shop to start following his true passion – farming.

"I have to keep moving son, gotta stay active," my father says.

"Not much to report on my end, Dad, busy with work as usual," I reply.

And then, after thinking about it for a moment, I ask: "Dad, you're 60 years old. Why did you decide to take up farming so late?"

After a beat, he responds: "It keeps me young. I'm outside with the chickens and a rooster. It's hard work, but I love it. Besides, if I didn't farm, I would either be dead of boredom or driving three hours a day to exercise with my son."

Which makes sense, I suppose.

"It's a little extreme, but I understand," I tell him. "When's the next time you're heading up our way for dinner and a glass of wine ... ?"

As you read through this book, I hope you understand how my parents and my clients have, and continue to inspire me personally and professionally. Seeing what they've been able to do was my motivation for writing this book.

So as you read through it, please remember that it's based on more than 10 years of professional experience, and the information in it is backed by reliable science and research.

Even more importantly, though, the contents of this book are based on firsthand observation of, and feedback from, clients who are over age 50 and have incorporated exercise into their lives. It tells their stories and how exercise has helped keep them vibrant, optimistic and enjoying life.

This book is about more than just motivation; it's a template to get you started, and most importantly, a call to action.

We don't have to do a lot; we've just got to do it right!

CHAPTER 1: PREPARING FOR RETIREMENT IS MORE THAN JUST FINANCIAL PLANNING

"Often when you think you're at the end of something, you're at the beginning of something else."

– Fred Rogers, longtime host of "Mister Rogers' Neighborhood"

I am 34 years old – nowhere close to even thinking about retiring. So who am I to be writing a book in which the first chapter is about planning for life after work? Good question.

I'm not a financial planner, a life coach or a lawyer. I'm a personal trainer with a degree in kinesiology. But, as a personal trainer, more than 70 percent of my clients are at least 50 years old – many much older – and more than two-thirds of them are retired. past decade, I've worked with many people who are thinking about retiring; who are newly retired; who are frustrated because, for one reason or another, they can't retire; or who have been retired for many years. So I've seen and heard a lot about retirement.

And, I've learned that everyone who retires has a different idea about what this next stage of their life should look like. Some people pursue the long-held interests they didn't have time for while working. Some travel to exotic locations, while others stay home and volunteer at the local school to help kids learn to read or deliver meals to homebound folks. Some hit the golf course with a vengeance, while others look forward to taking care of grandchildren.

When people retire, they generally have two big concerns: financial and fitness. They want to be comfortable enough financially to enjoy their retirement years, and fit and healthy enough to be able to do the things they enjoy.

If you're looking forward to, or already enjoying your retirement, it's likely that you've saved and invested wisely over the years. If that's the case, I commend you.

But, as important as your financial health is heading into retirement, your physical health is even more important.

Take a minute to picture your perfect retirement. Are you traveling? Gardening? Golfing for hours on end? None of those things can happen if you're physically inactive, unwell and spending your money and time on doctor visits and prescriptions. I guarantee the retirement you've planned for and fantasize about doesn't include continual hospital stays and afternoons spent at the physical therapy clinic.

Health is your most important asset. To put it into context, by exercising, you're investing and maintaining your asset, like saving or planning for your financial retirement. By continuing, or starting to exercise, you will be increasing and improving your longevity and quality of life.

If you compare your health to a car, what would your preference be? A high performance Mercedes or a 15-year-old clunker held together with duct tape and spit? That's a no-brainer.

Meet My Client: *The Admiral*

About five years ago, on the first day the Admiral decided to stop at our club, he turned off his car and sat in the parking lot. Finally, after thinking about it for a while, he showed up at the front desk.

"I almost didn't come in," he confessed. "I was very close to driving away."

"Thank you for stopping and trying us out," I said. "We treat exercise here like a swimming pool. Some people jump in off the deep end, and others dangle a toe in first, then the foot. However you want to start is OK. I'm not here to break you down; we're going to work to build you up."

The Admiral, a retired business owner, looked at me skeptically and said, "Let's give it a go."

The first week The Admiral began exercising, he started with the elliptical at low resistance. He lasted five minutes and was winded. He rested for a few moments, then continued. He completed 12 minutes on the elliptical that day.

"Slow and steady; this a marathon, not a sprint," I told him.

By the end of the month, the Admiral was completing 30-minute sessions on the elliptical six days a week at moderate to high intensity. During the first week of training, we had two strength training sessions.

"Learn the technique and movement pattern before adding speed or resistance to any of your exercises," I said.

"It's important for your body to learn the motor patterns -- train slow, play fast."

In the first couple of weeks, he did strength training twice a week, completing 4-6 resistance exercises per session. In two weeks, he was strength training three times a week, completing 8-10 strength exercises and we saw significant improvement in muscular strength, motor coordination and balance.

I asked him: "Hey Admiral, why at your age do you want to exercise? What was the light switch that clicked on? You've been retired for quite some time and you enjoy traveling, dining at fine restaurants, wine and attending sporting events. So, why?"

He looked at me with a puzzled expression, paused for a few seconds and said: "So, I can continue enjoying all those things you mentioned. And, it feels damn good to be stronger and more fit than someone who is 30 years younger."

True, the Admiral has excellent genes, but to remain that healthy at his age requires discipline and desire to maintain or improve health. At 81 years young, he is still sharp and still travels.

To this day, the Admiral continues to exercise. When he travels, he makes sure every hotel or resort has some form of a fitness center or one close by. Not too shabby for someone who almost never started his exercise journey.

Remember, it's never too late, and slow and steady al-

ways wins the race.

Investing in Your Future You

What if somebody told you there is something you can do every day that will reduce stress, improve some health and medical discomforts, keep health care costs under control and significantly improve your quality of life? Oh, and not to mention, slow the aging process.

Would you be interested?

What if I told you it was exercise? Simply starting to walk 30 minutes a day can make all the difference.

The reason I wanted to write this book is that I've seen too many loved ones affected by common health and medical issues that could have been easily prevented, or at least mitigated, by incorporating physical activity into their daily lives.

Think of exercise as an investment in improving or maintaining quality of life, enjoying the fruits of your labor and avoiding that 15-year-old clunker.

The Western world is becoming increasingly overweight, with more frequent incidences of cardiovascular diseases, Type 2 diabetes, orthopedic issues and Alzheimer's disease.

Here are some statistics that paint a picture of the current situation:

Only 34 percent of Americans over age 64 are physically active, making that demographic the most inactive of any.

About 65% of the major causes of death are lifestyle-related; further sedentary behavior is directly correlated with increased risk of cardiovascular disease.

Of the population 65 and older, 6.8 million people – or 25.2 percent -- are diagnosed with Type 2 diabetes (Medical News Today/2019).

Approximately 84 million Americans suffer from some form of cardiovascular disease. An estimated 33.9% of U.S. adults aged 18 years or older (84.1 million people) had prediabetes in 2015. Nearly half (48.3%) of adults aged 65 years or older had prediabetes (Centers for Disease Control and Prevention).

Being physically active doesn't need to be extreme. Most people working out today do so to stay healthy and fit; they're not slamming barbells to the floor, accompanied by loud grunts or war cries. Exercise today is more of a blue collar mentality. I like that.

Also, participating in physical exercise doesn't necessarily entail joining a gym or fitness studio. For most people, functional exercises can be incorporated daily from the comforts of home. Functional exercises are movement patterns (we will discuss later) that we utilize every day without even thinking about them.

In essence, your body is actually the gym. But doing a sit-up for your bowl of cheese curls or reaching for the TV remote doesn't count. You actually have to move, keep moving and build it into a habit.

That said, personal trainers and gyms do provide an advantage – accountability. Knowing that all the equipment is available, and someone is there waiting for you goes a long way in lighting a fire of motivation.

If you do choose to join a gym, you don't need to spend hours upon hours there. Depending on your medical limitations and health and fitness goals, your workout may only be 20-30 minutes, three times a week.

In fact, if you find yourself spending more than an hour in a gym, you're probably not sure where all the equipment is located (it happens), unclear about what exercise to do next (we will discuss later), or very busy socializing (which often can be a great thing).

Once you make up your mind that exercise is necessary – and yes, it is necessary and has to be completed today and every day -- we can take the next step of building a routine and becoming efficient in it.

Exercise: The Key to Successful Aging

I believe most people understand that it's better to remain physically and mentally active as they age. But that doesn't mean that most people stay active. I've seen way too many people resign themselves to thinking that physiological deterioration is inevitable with aging.

And here's what I'll tell you about that: It's not inevitable.

If you take one thing from this book, I hope it's the realization that you absolutely can remain strong, active and vibrant into your 70s, 80s and beyond. You can take control and slow – perhaps even turn back – the clock.

The over-50 clients I've trained have repeatedly demonstrated to me that exercise, when done regularly, has a positive effect and improves quality of life. Why would you not want that?

In my profession, things change all the time. There are always new ideas and updated research about exercising, how exercise should be delivered, how to train clients effectively and the effects of exercise on the body.

One thing that doesn't change is the idea that you've got to move. By moving, you send physiological signals through your body, telling it to keep developing and not break down. Once you start to move, your body will adapt quickly. It inherently understands that movement is survival and survival is movement.

It's true that I'm nowhere close to retirement age, but I have been in the health and fitness field for more than 10 years. In addition to my degree, I have continued with coursework and training, investing time, energy and knowledge to assure that I can train people safely and guide them toward their health and fitness goals. And, I've seen how adding even 10 minutes of movement to your daily routine can improve mobility and increase confidence.

The great majority of my clients aren't on a mission to compete physically or break any records. They're interested in exercising because they want to feel better, reduce aches and pains, improve their posture, reduce their risk of falling and be able to travel and play with their grandkids. Their goals aren't grandiose – just practical.

To Learn More

When learning a new skill, there are two processes we use to collect data: extrinsic learning and intrinsic learning.

Extrinsic learning is conscious learning and involves understanding instruction, technique and other intellectual insights. Intrinsic learning is experiential data gathered through our somatosensory system.

While both processes play an important role in skill acquisition, many athletes focus too much on the extrinsic stuff and ignore what their bodies are trying to tell them.

Check out this link to read more about how your body can talk to you. http://breakingmuscle.com/mobility-recovery/motor-control-and-movement-patterns-a-must-read-for-athletes

Exercise Equals Movement

For some, even mention of the word "exercise" is off-putting because they picture exercise as being laborious, sweaty and hard. I've had people scowl at me when I talk about exercise; looking at me like I've just said something totally inappropriate. And you know what? I get that. So, what if we'd use a different word for exercise?

Let's replace the word "exercise" with "movement." You move every single day, from the time you get up until bedtime. Everything we do during our daily routines involves one or more movement patterns. Basically, exercise is simply a series of movements with sets and repetitions.

There are five basic movements of human body: squat, hinge, press, pull and anti-rotational/rotational of the core.

It's amazing how variations of these five basic movements affect how we move throughout our day. These movements have made it possible for humans to survive, ever since we were hunter-gatherers. Each of these movement patterns is efficient and maximizes the human body's structure for speed, strength and agility.

The next time you're grocery shopping, carrying laundry up and down the stairs or shoveling snow, think about the movement pattern your body is employing.

To be clear, performing these basic movement patterns is not a substitute for exercise. Even if you walk around your office during your workday or climb the stairs instead of taking the elevator, you still have to exercise.

Consistently exercising will increase your energy level, making the day-to-day physical activities easier to accomplish. So even though the words "exercise" and "movement" will be used interchangeably in this book, don't mistake the action of moving about during your daily activities for a session of exercising.

Regardless of whether you're thinking about retiring, newly retired or have been settled into retirement life for years, getting into a routine of movement and exercise will help assure that you'll be at the top of your game and able to enjoy the years to come.

CHAPTER 2: A BRIEF HISTORY OF EXERCISE

"Since the time of the ancient Greeks, we have always felt that there was a close relationship between a strong, vital mind and physical fitness."

– John F. Kennedy, 35th President of the United States

My first interests may be kinesiology and fitness training, but I'm also a history enthusiast. So when I started contemplating how the societal concept of fitness has evolved and developed over time, I wanted to learn more about the history of exercise.

What I learned is that over the course of history, exercise has played vital roles in survival and nation building. Let me explain.

In prehistoric times, humans survived by hunting and gathering their food. They didn't stay in one place, but were constantly on the move, looking for seeds, fruit, nuts, small game and other forms of food.

A bit later, they learned to fish and created better tools that enabled them to track and kill bigger game. Life was based on finding enough food to survive, and finding food required constant movement to accommodate, among other things, changing seasons and shifting animal herds.

Exercise, however, was not limited to prehistoric humans.

The Persian Empire (550-330 BCE)

Physical activity was not only encouraged during this period, it was required of every son born under the empire, because the Persians realized the importance of building and developing soldiers who could defend the empire. Military personnel ranked high in the social structure of the Persian Empire, topped only by kings and priests.

Also, people of the Persian Empire built homes for themselves and constructed roadways. They wove clothing and rugs, and some were accomplished potters. Doing nothing was not an option.

The Ancient Greeks (2500-200 BCE)

In ancient Greece, development of the body was considered as important as development of the mind, resulting in citizens who were the epitome of exercise and fitness.

The ancient Greeks pursued physical perfection and sought to attain it through sports and activities, such as gymnastics, running, jumping and wrestling.

They established palestras, or gyms. The Paidotribes, or fitness trainers, were respected members of society. Ancient Greeks lived by the saying, "Exercise for the body, and music for the soul." Exercise and music were interwoven in daily life.

Sparta (900s-192 BCE)

Historians tell us that Sparta was quite possibly the most physically fit culture and society in the history of man. Spartans had a keen interest in exercise and fitness, primarily for military purposes.

Spartan men were professional soldiers, and those with the highest levels of fitness, strength and conditioning were most highly regarded in combat.

The Spartan zeal for fitness was even higher than that of the Athenians, which probably contributed to Sparta defeating Athens in the Peloponnesian War (431-404 BC).

Young males in Sparta began a rigorous training regimen as early as age 6 to assure they would mature into healthy and fit soldiers. Females were required to be physically fit as well, with the goal of bearing healthy, strong offspring.

Roman Civilization (200 BCE-476 CE)

According to some historians, the rise and fall of the Roman Empire parallels the rise and fall of the fitness of its people.

During Rome's period of empire building, the society was heavily invested in physical fitness and exercise. Roman males between ages 17 and 60 were eligible for the military draft and, in order to be prepared for combat, they had to be in peak physical condition. Military training consisted of activities such as running, marching, jumping and discus and javelin throwing.

The superior fitness of the Roman people resulted in Rome conquering nearly all of the Western world.

But after the expansion of the Roman Empire, the emphasis on physical activity declined significantly. Romans had acquired vast wealth and there was affluence throughout the empire.

The process of acquiring material goods and status pieces became priorities, and much of the population preferred entertainment, such as viewing gladiator battles, to physical exercise.

The lavish lifestyle and physical decay eventually took its toll as the Roman civilization fell to the physically superior Barbarian tribes from northern Europe.

Check This Out

Consider that over two centuries, the Roman army conquered England/Wales, Spain, Greece, France, parts of the Middle East and the northern coast of Africa. It's not surprising that physical prowess was not optional.

The Dark (476-1000 CE) and Middle Ages (900-1400 CE)

After the collapse of the Roman Empire, the known world experienced an intellectual stagnation. The affluent lifestyle epitomized during the Roman Empire was replaced with collective hardship for survival. People in this era reverted to being hunters, gatherers and foragers for survival; they were forced to stay physically active in order to survive. It is one of the few times that a "reset" of human civilization took place.

The Renaissance (1400-1600 CE)

The Renaissance, or "rebirth," was inspired and influenced by ancient Greek and Roman cultural learning. A renewed interest in fitness was due in part to renewed appreciation of the human body. The ancient Greeks and Romans highly valued the human anatomy.

Many individuals, including religious leader Martin Luther, philosopher John Locke and physical educators Vittorino da Feltra, John Comenius and Richard Mulcaster, believed that high fitness levels enhanced intellectual learning. As it was with the Greeks, exercise became an engrained way of life during the Renaissance.

United States – National Period (1776-1860 CE)

Not surprisingly, the Europeans influenced American culture during this early period of our country's history. Physical activity, such as gymnastics, was brought to the New World by German and Swedish immigrants, although it never reached the level of popularity it enjoyed in Europe.

Thomas Jefferson and Benjamin Franklin acknowledged the importance of exercise and physical activity, encouraging daily physical activity such as running, swimming and basic forms of resistance training to improve and maintain health.

Thought for the Day

"Not less than two hours a day should be devoted to exercise, and the weather shall be little regarded. If the body is feeble, the mind will not be strong."

– Thomas Jefferson, third President of the United States

Exercise has been prevalent throughout human history. Exercise and fitness were integral in building a better society and advancing civilization. The ancients, and even Colonial Americans, understood and shared this common view.

A population that was physically fit could gather food, farm, build, innovate and assure a strong military. In some cases, physical exercise and fitness were focal points for developing thought, philosophy and culture.

So here's the burning question: What happened?"

CHAPTER 3:
20TH CENTURY:
THE RISE OF
THE SEDENTARY
LIFESTYLE

"Take care of your body. It's the only place you have to live in."

– Jim Rohn, American businessman, author and motivational speaker

During the middle of the 20th century, a phenomenon regarding work and labor occurred in the United States: We started transitioning from predominantly physically demanding jobs (think steel mills, construction and farming) to jobs that were accomplished while sitting behind desks in offices.

For many people, that meant it was no longer necessary to maintain good physical condition in order accomplish their work. As more workers moved from the mills and mines to office jobs, their level of fitness decreased because they exercised less.

According to the Mayo Clinic, between 1970 and 2000, the number of workers in sedentary jobs doubled. And, with many of us having jobs that require little physical activity, our total screen time has increased dramatically. Even when we're not bound to a computer for work, many of us are spending our free time watching/streaming TV or glued to social media.

We also drive a lot, whether it's for business or getting the kids or grandkids from a piano lesson to soccer practice. It's estimated that the average person spends nearly four hours a day watching television and one hour driving. Overall, Americans sit for 13 hours every day, and sleep for six to eight hours a night.

That means the average American is active only three to five hours a day. And, by being active, we're not talking about running or strength training, biking or even walking; we're just talking about being up and moving about. That's a pretty startling statistic, don't you think?

Let's consider what happens to your body when you sit all day, whether it's at your desk, in front of your TV or on your front porch.

It doesn't take much time before your metabolism slows down. Muscles start to get tight, posture compromises and flexibility and range of motion are out the window. Typically, as the average person's metabolism slows, the consumption of calories and the volume of food do not. As a result, gradual weight gain ensues.

Sitting for long periods of time also creates significant blood pooling in the lower extremities, which makes it harder for the cardiovascular system to run efficiently. As your muscles stiffen and weaken, posture is affected, and it becomes difficult to support your increased body weight.

Eventually, you may experience an upper and/or lower cross syndrome. With the upper cross, the shoulders roll forward, the upper back is stiff and rounded, the neck protrudes forward and the chest caves in.

With the lower cross, the abdomen is weakened, the lower back muscles and hip flexors shorten and stiffen, and the glutes are weakened. Either of these syndromes can affect balance, range of motion and flexibility.

Your mind and body are continually collecting feedback from your environment. If you are not moving for the vast majority of your day, your mind and body will adapt accordingly. At the end of the day, you're not fatigued from hard work; your body and mind are tired from being sedentary.

Our changes in lifestyle have yielded some troubling results:

One in three people in the United States is obese.

One in three is hypertensive.

One in10 is diabetic.

Clearly, our bodies suffer when repeatedly seated for extended periods of time. Medical professionals compared sedentary workers, such as bus drivers, to those who are continuously on the move, such as trash collectors, and found that the seated workers have a significantly higher chance of developing Type 2 diabetes and cardiovascular disease.

Check This Out

A 2016 study by the American Cancer Society and the National Cancer Institute revealed that regular exercise lowers the risk of 13 types of cancer, including colon, breast, endometrial, esophageal, stomach, and liver. That's pretty good incentive to move, isn't it?

I have not presented this information to make you feel guilty or bad about your lifestyle. I'm not assigning fault for today's style of living, which is a result of a complicated set of circumstances.

The way we work has changed. Certain technologies encourage inactivity. Safety concerns prohibit many children from unrestricted outdoor activity and discourage adults from exercising outside. We have greater access to less healthy foods. The list goes on and on.

The point is, being sedentary for the majority of the day is counterintuitive and has become an enemy to our health. We need to find a balance regarding work, activity and rest. We need to rethink the amounts of time we spend being sedentary compared to the time we spend moving.

So, what does that look like? How can we mitigate this problem of inactivity?

Step 1: Avoid being seated for longer than one hour at a time. Try to stand up and walk for a bit every 20 minutes.

Step 2: Exercise regularly. An additional 30-minute walk and some strength training will prevent wear and tear on the body.

Step 3: Stretch. Flexibility in the skeletal muscles promotes blood flow throughout the tissues as well as elasticity, which prevents muscle stiffness and shortening.

To quote the Mayo Foundation for Medical Education and Research:

"Compared with our parents or grandparents, we are spending increasing amounts of time in environments that not only limit physical activity, but require prolonged sitting – at work, at home, and in our cars and communities.

"Work sites, schools, homes and public spaces have been (and continue to be) re-engineered in ways that minimize human movement and muscular activity. These changes have a dual effect on human behavior: People move less and sit more. From an evolutionary perspective, humans were designed to move -- and engage in all manner of manual labor throughout the day. This was essential to our survival as a species. The recent shift from a physically demanding life to one with few physical challenges has been sudden, occurring during a tiny fraction of human existence."

This quote by Lance C. Dalleck, M.S. and Len Kravitz, Ph.D., authors of *"The History of Exercise,"* says it all; *"It appears that as societies become too enamored with wealth, prosperity and self-entertainment that fitness levels drop. In addition, as technology has advanced with man, the levels of physical fitness have decreased."*

In our current circumstances, with unprecedented rates of obesity, preventable diseases and a declining life expectancy nationwide, I think it's safe to say that, once again, the primary purpose of exercise has become survival.

Meet my Client: Linda

"So, why do you exercise and stay physically active?" I asked my client, Linda, who is 64 and preparing to retire in the spring.

She told me she started exercising 10 years previously, when her father was diagnosed with heart disease. She recognized her risk of heart disease and knew it was important for her to take care of herself.

I've been working with Linda for more than three years and she is one of the most physically fit clients I've ever had. Her commitment to exercise will not only help her avoid heart disease, but also allow her to fully enjoy an active and busy retirement.

Linda enjoys traveling, visiting art museums, shopping for antiques, gardening and exploring new cities. Thanks to her habit of daily exercise and other positive habits, she's able to do all those things and to look forward to a long and healthy life.

Current Trend of Exercise and Physical Activity Participation

Let's take a closer look at what's going on in our country as it relates to exercise and fitness trends and statistics.

According to the Physical Activity Council (PAC), a national organization that annually partners with sports, fitness and recreation associations to determine participation levels, except for the very elderly, the Baby Boomer generation (those born between 1945 and 1964) is the most inactive group of Americans. One third of this demographic participates in no type of intentional exercise.

The Centers for Disease Control and Prevention (CDC) in 2013 published a research study concluding that nearly 80 percent of the U.S. population 18 years and older, does not complete the recommended amounts of exercise each week, which puts that group in a position for future health related problems.

According to a CBS News report, the CDC recommends adults get at least 2.5 hours of moderate-intensity aerobic exercise or 75 minutes of vigorous-intensity activity, or a combination of both each week. Adults should also engage in muscle-strengthening activities such as lifting weights or doing push-ups at least twice a week.

Another CBS News report indicated that, according to Harvard researchers, inactivity is linked to 5.3 million deaths worldwide, similar to the number of deaths linked to smoking.

Lack of physical activity is not just a problem for the Baby Boomers, but also Gen Xers (born between mid-1960s and early 1980s), Millennials (born between 1977 and 1994) and Gen Z's (born between 1995 and 2012), as well.

But it's not only age that determines who exercises and who doesn't. Social status, income, where you live and level of education also are factors.

I could go on about the lack of physical activity in America, but suffice it to say that, while most people agree that exercising is necessary for a healthy life, the majority of those people don't exercise.

A major problem is that younger people learn about exercise habits and attitudes toward fitness from older people, which means that many of us may need to rethink our own attitudes and habits if we want to positively influence those who come after us.

CHAPTER 4: MYTHS ABOUT AGING, AND WHY THEY'RE NOT TRUE

"Of all the self-fulfilling prophecies in our culture, the assumption that aging means decline and poor health is probably the deadliest."

–Marilyn Ferguson, American author and public speaker

The dilemma is that you either get old, or you don't. Most of us, I'm assuming, would choose the former over the latter. The challenge, then, is to grow old while maintaining optimal health and fitness levels. And, that is completely possible.

The human body is an incredible piece of engineering. Highly adaptable and malleable, your body adjusts to and strengthens with activity. When you exercise, your central nervous system (CNS) acts like computer hardware, gathering and interpreting data from your movements and activities. As you continue to exercise, your CNS adapts to the new information it's receiving and becomes more efficient as your strength increases.

Of course, that works the opposite way, as well. When you're not active, your body adjusts to that, too, resulting in a slowed metabolism, weight gain, aches, stiffness, joint pain and decreased muscular strength -- none of which are any fun.

As we age, our bodies tend to lose some of their plasticity and start to become a bit rigid. You still possess the muscle-skeletal, circulatory and neurological properties to adapt and overcome, it's just that the ability to adapt takes longer. It's like switching from a cable modem to dial-up internet: You can still access the web, but you'll need to be patient.

Staying physically active and exercising regularly can assure that you maintain muscle-skeletal strength and, if your exercise routine has been minimal or lacking, your strength will significantly increase as you age.

It's true that our bodies experience dramatic physiological changes as we age, and your strength at 50 or 60 might not be what it was when you were 30. But that doesn't mean that you're not able to remain active and vital.

Individuals who accept and embrace the aging process are more likely to maintain a positive attitude and be able to take the necessary steps to stay healthy and turn back the clock on aging. They don't buy into myths of aging. There are lots of variations on "myths of aging," but here are my top five. Let's take a look and discover why they are just that ... myths.

Myth No. 1: Becoming Fragile and Brittle is Inevitable

As a health and fitness professional, this is the No. 1 myth I encounter when working with a client over 60.

The human body becomes fragile for different reasons, namely, physical inactivity, poor diet, genetics and poor lifestyle choices, such as excessive alcohol consumption and sedentary behavior.

Developing and maintaining a physically active lifestyle with daily exercise and proper eating will keep you moving and fit. Muscular strength training and a weight-bearing, cardio-respiratory activity, such as walking, will increase your muscular strength and improve your balance, reducing the risk of osteoporosis and fractures.

Adopting a physically active lifestyle enables you to fight back against the tide of aging and its physiological maladies. By exercising and eating properly, you are being proactive and entering the aging process on your own terms, which is a boost to self-confidence and self-esteem.

The concept of brittle and fragile is an afterthought in those who remain physically active in aging.

Myth No. 2: Old Age Kills Libido and Sex Drive

Old age does not kill libido and sex drive, but multiple physiological and psychological factors directly affect the sex drive in aging individuals. Those who don't take care of their health or maintain an active physical lifestyle certainly have an increased chance of decreased libido and sexual appetite.

Individuals over 50 who have already been diagnosed with a cardiovascular or metabolic disease are especially likely to experience a compromised libido.

Hypertension and atherosclerosis (a buildup of plaque in the arteries) have a significant negative effect on sexual activity due to cardiovascular restriction. Other chronic diseases or pain also can affect desire and ability to have or enjoy sex.

Psychological factors also affect sex drive. Those who don't feel attractive or experience poor self-esteem or self-confidence are likely to be negatively affected, as are people who suffer from depression, have experienced trauma or are impacted by other emotional or psychological issues.

So, it's not old age that kills libido or sex drive; it's an individual's physical and psychological health. Maintaining exercise and physical activity can improve health and help assure you can enjoy sex well into your 70s, 80s or beyond!

To Learn More

You can learn more about sex and aging at:

http://www.ncbi.nlm.nih.gov/pmc/articles/ PMC3267340/

http://www.ncbi.nlm.nih.gov/pmc/articles/ PMC3349920/

http://www.nytimes.com/2007/04/10/ health/10brod.html?_r=0

Myth No. 3: You Will Lose Your Independence as You Age

While some older adults do experience a loss of independence caused by a variety of factors, others remain active and on their own for their entire lives.

Factors that affect how long a person is able to maintain independence include lifestyle, genetics, cognitive skills, nutrition and physical and mental activity. This book focuses on physical activity and aging, but mental activity is just as important.

Reading, learning a new language, taking a course and social interactions are great ways to put yourself through a mental workout.

I cannot stress enough the importance of an active daily lifestyle. Your continued independence will be directly related to how well you can move or not move. The ability to navigate steps, complete chores and take care of your personal needs is vital to your continued independence.

Aging does not take our independence; we lose it by not taking care of our health and wellness. Incorporating strength training, cardiovascular workouts and exercises to increase balance, flexibility, mobility and stability into your weekly schedule will reduce the chances of losing your independence as you age.

To Learn More

You can learn more about maintaining functional independence at: http://gerontologist.oxfordjournals.org/content/42/1/24.full

Myth No. 4: Older People Should Limit Physical Activity

Yes, your physical activity probably will decrease as you age -- but just slightly. You most likely won't lift as much or run as fast when you're in your 50s as you did in your 20s, but that doesn't mean you should stop lifting and running, or at least walking. By all means, you should exercise and stay physically active within your limits to physiologically turn back the aging clock.

Thought for the Day

"What you think you are, you become. What you feel, you attract. What you imagine, you create."

– Gautama Buddha, founder of Buddhism

Physical limitations are boundaries that affect individuals with poor or compromised health. Incorporating an active daily lifestyle can keep those limitations at bay, and even expand the amount of physical activity you're able to accomplish.

I have clients in their 60s, 70s and 80s who are more physically active than some people I know in their 20s and 30s. They accomplish that high level of activity by setting goals, maintaining busy schedules and continuing to move.

Myth No. 5: The Amount of Sleep You Need Decreases with Age

Sleep is just as important in your 50s, 60s and beyond as it was when you were 30. We know, however, that physiological changes are normal as we age, and sleep patterns often change.

Studies show that many older people have trouble falling asleep and experience increased sleep fragmentation, which is interruption to normal sleep patterns. Physiological and psychological disorders and some medications also can increase sleep fragmentation.

In addition, older people tend to become sleepier in the early evening and wake earlier in the morning compared to younger adults. This is due to changes in the circadian rhythms that coordinate the timing of our bodily functions, including sleep.

The sleep rhythm is shifted forward so that you'll still end up sleeping for seven or eight hours; you'll just go to sleep earlier at night and wake up earlier in the morning. Your old midnight to 7 a.m. schedule changes to a 10 p.m. to 5 or 6 a.m. schedule.

To Learn More

You can learn more about sleep patterns in older adults and get tips for sleeping better at:

https://sleepfoundation.org/sleep-topics/aging-and-

sleep

https://www.sleepfoundation.org/articles/healthy-sleep-tips

Obviously, the amount of sleep needed varies from person to person. The optimum range, as recommended by the National Sleep Foundation, is between seven and nine hours a night for adults.

If you are experiencing a lot of trouble sleeping, you should consult your primary care provider. If you often are jolted out of sleep or have trouble with excessive snoring, you should discuss the possibility of sleep apnea with your doctor.

Practicing positive sleep hygiene helps, as well. Make sure your room is quiet and dark, and that you're not distracted by electronics or television. And of course, regular exercise and a good diet also are beneficial in improving sleep.

Hopefully, debunking these myths about aging will make you feel a little less anxious and more confident about your ability to age well. By maintaining your best level of fitness -- physically and psychologically -- you'll increase the odds of achieving the lifestyle you hope for.

Everyone deserves a happy, productive and graceful aging process, but you need to be willing to work to make that happen.

Research tells us that even 30 minutes of moderate exercise a day can help prevent chronic diseases, keep your weight under control, help you maintain flexibility and improve your psychological outlook.

That doesn't seem like too much to ask, does it?

Meet My Client: Ms. Peggy

Meet Ms. Peggy, a 73-year-old client who I've been working with for more than two years. Five years before we started working together, when Peggy was 66, she suffered a severe shoulder injury in which she shattered the head of the humerus and shoulder socket. After a complete shoulder reconstruction, she was slightly depressed due to the lack of range of motion in the joint and the effect it had on her day-to-day activities. She experienced constant pain and throbbing throughout the day, which made gardening, running and horseback riding – all activities she had enjoyed -- difficult.

We came up with a disciplined exercise regimen that incorporated strength training, flexibility, range of motion, balance and motor coordination tasks. Peggy has been able to significantly improve the function of her shoulder, which has given her more independence and freedom, basically improving her quality of life.

Keep in mind, she is now 75 years young, proving that we can absolutely change and turn our lives around if we want to. I find her story to be incredible, because it's a great example of how maintaining a disciplined routine and mindset can make all the difference. Peggy recently decided she wanted to retire -- key word being "decided". She now enjoys her afternoons working in the garden, exercising and, at the end of the day, a delicious micro-brew.

In the next chapter, we'll look at what typically occurs physiologically as we age. And, we'll see how exercising and staying active can slow or even prevent those changes.

CHAPTER 5: THE CRUCIAL ROLE OF EXERCISE IN MAINTAINING PHYSICAL, MENTAL AND EMOTIONAL HEALTH IN AGING

"If you are in a bad mood go for a walk. If you are still in a bad mood, go for another walk."

- Hippocrates, Greek physician

When done with some thought, determination, luck and a bit of grace, aging can be a rewarding and exciting process.

Chances are that you're better off financially than you were a few decades ago, and hopefully enjoying the fruits of your labor. Many 50-plus folks I work with find that they're better able to cope with setbacks than they once were -- a reward of maturity and life experience.

Aging can bring with it opportunities for enjoying activities you didn't previously have time for. Perhaps you're able to do some traveling, spend time with your grandkids, volunteer for a cause or explore a new hobby.

But in order to reap the benefits and rewards that are encountered later in life, you'll need to assure that you're in the best condition possible -- physically, mentally and emotionally. And, that means that you'll need to exercise.

When you become overly stressed, don't eat or sleep well, are not physically active and don't maintain important social connections, your mind and body are negatively affected, which also plays a role in your emotional health.

There's plenty of research that links the connectedness of those aspects of health. When our physical, mental or emotional health suffers, other aspects of health suffer, as well.

To Learn More

This book primarily deals with staying physically fit, which also benefits your mental and emotional health. Another way of staying healthy, according to a study from Stanford University, is to maintain social connections.

You can read more about that at http:// ccare.stanford.edu/uncategorized/connectedness-health-the-science-of-social-connection-infographic/

Caring for your entire being helps to assure that you'll remain physically strong, mentally sharp and emotionally balanced. Sure, there are no guarantees. People get sick or develop dementia or encounter a life circumstance with which they simply can't cope.

But by minding all aspects of your health, you can greatly increase the odds of aging successfully and happily.

Physical Benefits of Exercise

As we age, most of us will experience decreased muscle strength and bone mass, weight gain and an increase in percentage of body fat. Muscles and connective tissue become stiff and inflexible, and reaction time slows significantly.

If you're thinking that's not great news, you're right. It's not great news. The great news is that, while physical aging is inevitable -- except for the alternative, which is that you don't live long enough to get old -- it can be slowed from a sprint to a crawl.

And that, of course, happens with regular exercise. There is a fountain of youth, but it isn't in Florida (of all places), as Ponce de Leon imagined. It's located in your gym, next to your exercise bike or in places along your neighborhood walking route.

In the next three chapters, you'll read about getting started with an exercise program, the types of exercises you'll want to do and the benefits of working with a trainer.

For now, let's go over what happens to your body when you exercise regularly and sustain that exercise routine for two years or longer. Basically, you will experience a physiological reset.

You will lose excess body weight. This is important because we know that losing even a small percentage of your overall body weight can result in significant improvements in blood pressure, cholesterol and blood sugar levels.

Your blood-glucose regulation improves, making it less likely that you'll develop Type 2 diabetes.

Your balance and motor coordination skills improve, making it less likely that you'll fall.

Your bone mass increases, making it less likely that you'll break a bone in the event that you do fall.

Your muscles will get stronger and your endurance will increase, meaning you'll have a lot more energy and ability to do things like helping to build a tree house for a grandchild or trekking through the Swiss Alps.

Your blood pressure will maintain or decrease, making you less reliant on medications and decreasing your risk of heart attack or stroke.

Cholesterol and triglyceride levels will improve, lowering your risk of atherosclerosis, a form of heart disease.

Once you've established and maintained a consistent exercise routine, your mind and body start to find a new "set point." In other words, if you are overweight and incorporate positive lifestyle habits, your body will begin to drop the excess body weight.

Once you've shed the pounds, your mind and body will establish a new baseline to maintain your decreased body weight. Through consistent exercise and maintenance of a healthy diet, your body will determine a set point and you'll tend to maintain that more healthy weight.

Crash dieting, on the other hand, inevitably results in gaining lost weight back, because the body doesn't have time to establish a new set point and reverts to the established point.

People who lose and regain weight time after time

actually end up with net weight gain; plus, it becomes increasingly difficult to lose weight again.

Losing weight in a methodical, gradual and consistent manner gives your body time to establish a new set point and reduces the chance that you'll regain the weight.

Sure, the scale might tip upwards after a couple of weeks of holiday parties, but maintaining your weight within a narrow range of pounds is much healthier than wide swings in weight.

Thought for the Day

When working with clients, I constantly stress the importance of consistency. Exercise should be as consistent as your morning cup of coffee. You need consistency to reach a healthy place and consistency to stay there. Establishing a habit of exercise is half the battle, whether it's a daily 30-minute walk or three or four days a week exercising at the gym.

Emotional and Mental Benefits of Exercise

You've read about how your body ages physically, and about the connection between your physical, mental and emotional health.

While it's important to take care of your body by exercising, eating well, getting enough sleep and having regular check-ins with your doctor, being attuned to your emotional and mental health is equally important.

Just as your body does, your brain changes as you age. A characteristic of the brain, just like the body, is plasticity, which reduces over time. That reduces the ability of your brain to adapt to and overcome the challenges of life. You might find that as you age it takes longer to complete cognitive tasks, or that you have more trouble remembering where you left your car keys.

Older people also are more likely to experience depression and anxiety than younger folks, although with increasing rates among young people these days, it seems as if there is plenty of depression and anxiety to go around.

Fortunately, there's a way to slow the changes that affect the brain, and I'll bet you can guess what it is. Of course, it's exercise.

Exercise among older people provides psychological benefit as well as physical, especially regular exercise routines conducted over a long period of time.

Maintaining cognitive function, which includes memory, decision-making skills, ability to learn, attention, goal setting and problem solving, is vital to healthy aging.

Regular exercise can help you do that. In the short term, it increases your ability to relax, reduces stress and anxiety and enhances your mood.

In the long term, it results in an overall sense of well-being, stronger self-esteem, self-efficacy and greater sense of control over your life; it helps manage mental conditions such as depression and anxiety; and it may help delay certain age-related cognitive declines.

Exercising -- physically and mentally – keeps us healthier than not exercising. So, why not get moving? Your physical, mental and emotional health depend on it.

Thought for the Day

While we normally think of exercise as a physical endeavor, mental exercise is just as important. Mental exercises to help maintain cognitive function could include learning a new language and practicing it on a trip or reading challenging books that broaden your vocabulary and force you to consider varying viewpoints.

You could take a course online or at an area academic institution. Or, get into the habit each evening of mentally reviewing every conversation you had that day. That not only sharpens memory, it gives you a chance to evaluate and follow up on subject matter.

Moving On

We've covered a lot of material in these first five chapters. You've learned about the importance and benefits of exercise, along with a little bit about the way lifestyle and exercise have changed over the centuries.

You've read about five myths of aging and how caring for yourself through regular exercise and other good habits can help you to debunk those myths.

So, with all that information in mind, let's get down to business and get you kicking some butt with an exercise routine that works for the fitness level you're at right now.

In the next chapter, you'll learn about getting started in an exercise program, which is really important if you've been inactive for a while.

Chapter 7 goes over some specific exercises that will be beneficial to your workout and illustrates how to do them properly and avoid injury, because nobody needs a pulled hamstring or an aching knee.

In Chapter 8, you'll read about gym basics, the benefits of getting some help from a trainer, and what to look for and ask if you decide to go that route.

So, thanks for hanging in for the first five chapters. Now let's get started – together!

CHAPTER 6: GETTING STARTED – IT'S NOT AS HARD AS YOU THINK

"And in the end, it's not the years in your life that count. It's the life in your years."

- Abraham Lincoln, 16th President of the United States

So, you're feeling committed to getting active (or more active) and into a regular exercise schedule. Trust me, that's great news. But if you haven't been a regular exerciser, it's likely that you have a lot of questions about what you should be doing to establish good habits, how you might feel when you first get started and how to set reasonable goals.

In this chapter, you'll get answers to all of those questions and more, as well as a lot of advice and information. Here we go!

Check in with Your Doctor

If you haven't worked out in more than two years, or you're not sure about your current health status, I strongly recommend that you see your primary care provider for a check-up to make sure that everything is in working order.

During the physical, tell your doctor that you want to start a physical activity program. He or she will give you a thumbs-up or down to begin.

This a big step to clear. The physical will give you feedback regarding when and how to start your exercise program, and how much you may be able to do at first. It also should provide you with some peace of mind regarding your current health status and give you a chance to ask questions and address any concerns you might have.

And, it will give you and/or your personal trainer a baseline of where to safely begin exercising. Once you've been checked out and cleared for action, you can put that fantastic muscle machine to work.

Fit Tip

Most healthcare providers operate on tight schedules, with limited time for each patient. Consider using a patient portal or email to convey any questions or concerns you have in advance of your appointment.

On Your Own or with a Trainer?

Your journey can proceed in one of two ways: You can venture out on your own, or you can work with a personal trainer (strongly recommended, especially if you've never exercised or lack motivation).

While venturing out on your own is not necessarily a bad idea, keep in mind that you definitely will experience a trial-and-error period. For example, you'll have to determine what exercises to do, the number of reps, the amount of resistance that's appropriate and what type and how much cardio is best.

By working with a fitness professional, you can significantly shorten that trial-and-error period.

Meeting with a knowledgeable health and fitness

professional is not just for inexperienced exercisers. Everyone at some point should meet and discuss their health and fitness goals with a high-quality, recommended professional.

If you were investing hard-earned money into a retirement plan or stock portfolio, you could go it alone, and probably become proficient in the process after a while. But think about how much time and effort you could save by consulting with a professional financial advisor. And chances are, your money will perform better when handled by an expert.

By researching different firms, talking to friends and meeting with different advisors, you will find someone who knows where to invest your money.

The same process can be used for choosing a gym and a trainer to help you with a more important investment than your money – your health.

Fighting Inertia

Once you're checked in with your doctor and established whether to work with a trainer or go it alone, the next step in getting off to a great start is learning how to fight inertia. It takes a lot of mental energy to make a new task part of your daily routine, but with exercising, it's well worth the effort.

It's no different than the habit of brushing your teeth every morning. Once you make exercising a daily habit, it becomes a task that must be completed every day. Noticing physiological improvements along your exercising journey – improved muscular strength, taking the stairs without getting winded, increased energy level – will motivate you to keep going.

Thought for the Day

Studies have shown that it takes three weeks to establish a routine. If you're just getting started, begin by setting a schedule and exercising for 30 minutes three days a week. After three weeks, the routine will be locked in and you can think about adding a fourth day. Do four days for three weeks and add a fifth day. By designating your exercise time on your calendar and keeping a record of your accomplishments, you'll stay on track as you move toward your goals.

Setting Goals

Goal setting is absolutely essential when you're beginning to exercise. I always say that setting personal health and fitness goals requires three elements: reality, practicality and a sprinkle of loftiness. Your goals will be the checkpoints on your journey to turning back the clock.

Establishing down-to-earth goals gives you concrete destination points in the immediate short term and medium term. The sprinkle of loftiness, which is a destination point that's slightly out of reach but ultimately attainable, is useful in establishing your long-term goal.

Should your lofty goal be running a 40-yard dash in 4.3 seconds? Well, no. But, doing yard work, gardening for four or five hours or playing 18 holes of golf? Absolutely!

Short-term vs. Long-term Goals

Goals can be short or long term, but be sure they're realistic. Losing 50 pounds or gaining 10 pounds of muscle in a month is not realistic.

A short-term goal could be dropping a pants size in three months, losing five pounds in a month or exercising for 30 minutes, three times a week for two months.

Examples of long-term goals might be to effectively improve your eating habits over the course of a year or losing 50 pounds over two years.

Once you've determined your short- and long-term goals, write them down and post them where you'll see them often. Doing that makes your goals concrete.

By concentrating on your short-term versus your long-term goals, your journey to a healthier you becomes more attainable and less overwhelming.

That's important, because focusing on long-term goals can lead to frustration and ultimately giving up. It's easy to lose your motivation when making a lifestyle change, so focus on short-term goals and going one day at a time.

Fit Tip

Footwear technology and design has progressed significantly over the past 10 years. So be sure to invest in appropriate shoes. We tend to forget that our feet are the only point of contact to the ground. If your shoes don't provide the right cushion, support and traction, you have a higher risk of injury, and may be less likely of developing an exercise routine. It's definitely worth getting your gait and foot analyzed prior to investing in a pair of shoes for exercise.

Recognizing Setbacks

On this journey to a healthier you, there will be slip-ups and even minor setbacks. It happens, or should I say, "Life happens.

Remember, you're committed for the long haul. If you miss a day of exercising because you need to take the grandkids to their piano recital, no worries. Hit the gym that evening or go first thing the next day.

Changing your lifestyle requires time and commitment. Ultimately, though, you must believe that it's worth the effort. Just remember that old saying, "Keep your eyes on the prize," which, in this case, is improved health.

Understanding Health and Fitness Goals

The first thing to understand is that health and fitness goals are very different. The No. 1 rule of exercise is that you do it first to improve your health, then your fitness.

Think about this: Your health is like the roots of a tree. It keeps you upright and strong. Your fitness is the solid trunk of that tree that can't grow without strong roots.

So health goals – lowering blood pressure, improving blood-glucose regulation and losing weight – can increase your quality of life and reduce your mortality risk.

Fitness goals, on the other hand, might be bench pressing your body weight or running a 5K.

Both health and fitness goals are important, and meeting fitness goals can be rewarding and confidence boosting. But you can complete a 5K or bench press your body weight and still not be healthy.

Incorporating a comprehensive training program

that addresses your health concerns, while at the same time moving you toward your fitness goals, is the ultimate solution.

Knowing What to Expect

If you haven't been physically active or exercised frequently, you can expect to experience some muscle soreness when you begin a fitness program. That, believe or not, is a good thing. While muscle soreness shouldn't be a deterrent to exercise, the "no pain, no gain" adage is not applicable to improving your health. You want to push yourself, but not hurt yourself.

Sometimes soreness results from slight tears in the skeletal muscle tissue. Wait, what, tears? Yes, but that only means that it's giving your body a chance to adapt by growing stronger muscle fibers.

If you experience soreness, try to keep exercising and maintain your routine. The feeling will subside. The goal is to be slightly sore, not incapacitated.

During the first two weeks of regular exercise, you probably will experience a lack of energy and feel a bit fatigued. Again, this is normal as your body adapts to the extra workload and energy expenditure. Once that happens, your energy level should improve significantly.

You also might experience a slight weight gain due

to inflammation. When tissues such as skeletal muscles break down, inflammation occurs to help heal the soft tissue. This is temporary and will stop as your body adapts to the physical activity.

Hopefully, the information in this chapter has been useful and motivating. Just remember that starting anything new can be daunting. Ask for help when you need it and don't beat yourself up if you don't immediately accomplish what you think you should be able to do.

The important thing is that you've taken the first steps to improving your health and getting and staying fit.

CHAPTER 7: ESTABLISHING A ROUTINE ... LESS IS MORE

"Once you are doing exercise regularly, the hardest thing is to stop it."

– Erin Gray, American actress

If you've identified short- and long-term goals for your health and fitness journey, you've completed an important first step. If you haven't identified goals yet, that's OK. They will become clear as you work your way through the rest of this book. For now, I want to talk about building a routine.

One word that's used all the time in my house is "consistency."

This magical word is the difference between success and failure when you're working on establishing a lifestyle change. Consistency is the wet cement that solidifies into a routine.

Once you've identified and established your goals, completing the day-to-day tasks will result in significant benefit to you. But to do that, you'll need to resist looking for instant gratification and focus on the long-term objective that is your goal. Yes, you'll achieve that long-term objective by meeting a series of short-term goals, but don't lose sight of the big picture.

Fit Tip

Be assured that there's nothing wrong with starting and building an exercise program at your own pace. Even 10 or 15 minutes of activity for someone who's been inactive for a long time is a great start. The key is to be relentless about building a routine and staying consistent.

A strategy that has always worked for me is to establish a baseline routine, say, walking on a treadmill for 20 minutes every day. Once you're in the habit of doing that, add two minutes or five minutes or whatever makes sense to you. Once you're in the habit of walking 22 or 25 minutes every day, add several more minutes. This allows you to build up your workout gradually, while establishing consistency in your routine.

Once your routine is well established and has become a habit, you can go a step further. Take a good look at your daily habits and be honest about those things that are not benefiting your physical, mental or spiritual health. Maybe you need to stop obsessing over CNN and start reading again. Or trade in the afternoon cookies for a bowl of fruit. But don't try to do these things while you're still in the process of building a consistent exercise routine. Small steps equal miles walked in the end.

Start with the Basics

Let's start by reviewing some basic exercises that should become part of your routine. You don't need to do every exercise every day, especially when you're just starting. Completing three exercises per session is a great start.

The exercises we're going to review incorporate movements that you use every day during your normal activities, without even thinking about them: squat, hinge, lunge, push, pull, core rotation and anti-rotation.

While performing exercises isn't rocket science, you should use caution and be aware that doing them incorrectly can make you susceptible to injury. If you've never exercised, or it's been a very long time, I strongly recommend starting with a health and fitness professional who can help you with form and in establishing a routine.

A Matter of Balance

Many people find that their sense of balance is affected as they age, caused by factors such as loss of muscle strength, reduced flexibility, nerve damage in the lower legs, use of certain medications and inner ear problems. This is something that can, and certainly should be addressed, as a loss of balance or impaired balance can significantly increase the likelihood of falls, which are the major cause of fractures among the older population. These simple exercises can significantly improve your balance.

Single Leg Balance Exercise:

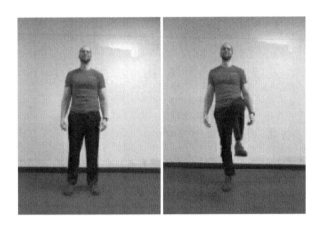

Half- Squat with Eyes Closed Balance Exercise:

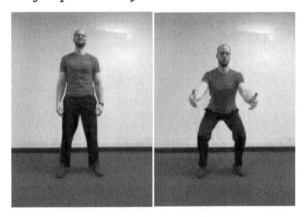

Squats

This is a movement pattern we do every day and it involves more than 200 skeletal muscles. Squats are a knee dominant movement, compared with the hinge movement, which is a hip dominant. The squat utilizes all three planes of motion and is the most metabolically demanding movement of the six listed above.

The squat is typically executed by having both feet hip width apart, toes slightly pointed out, and feet flat on the floor. While maintaining upright posture, begin to lower your body toward the floor by flexing at the ankles, knees and hips. The depth of your squat is determined by pain-free range of motion and where you can maintain balance.

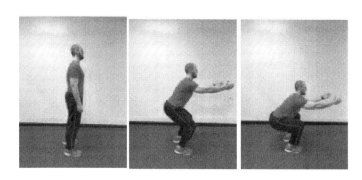

Hinges

The hinge pattern is a powerful movement. The hips generate a tremendous amount force, whether you're playing a sport, dancing or picking up grandkids or groceries from the floor. As a hip dominant pattern, the rest of the body remains stable while your hips create the movement. Start this movement with your feet hip width apart and a slight knee bend. Maintaining the starting position, push your butt back like you're trying to knock someone over. This movement is created by your hips and not the low back.

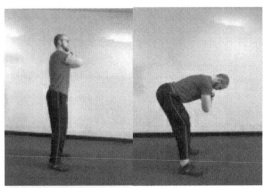

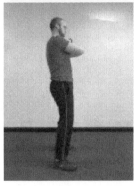

Lunges (step or walking)

The lunge is the third of the lower-body-focused movements. The lunge requires that the legs are in a split position, one foot forward and one foot back, and both feet are hip width apart. You want the back leg positioned so that the knee is behind the hip, the ankle behind the knee, and the back foot on its toes. The front foot is flat. Once in position, both knees flex, lowering the body to the floor. The depth of your lunge is determined by pain-free range of motion and your ability to maintain balance.

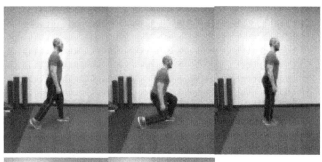

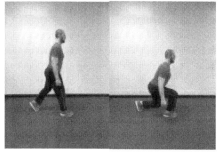

Push

The push pattern is our most utilized movement. If you work at a desk, drive a car, cook, move a shopping cart or even use the remote control, you're employing the push pattern. All of those examples require you to push away from your body. Pushing exercises include the chest press, shoulder press and push-up. Most of us, unfortunately, perform too many pushing and not enough pulling exercises. That imbalance creates postural issues like the upper cross syndrome or problems with the rotator cuff and neck.

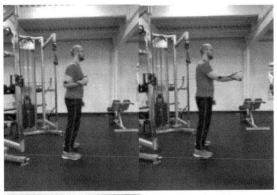

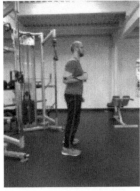

Pull

The pull pattern is probably the most underutilized movement in everyday life. Due to sedentary behavior, technology, work (seated at a desk ALL DAY) and leisure activities (seated on a comfy couch ALL DAY), the muscles that create the push pattern get a workout, while those that create the pull pattern remain largely unused. When the pull pattern becomes weak or inefficient, it can compromise your posture and create shoulder and neck problems. As mentioned in the section above, imbalance in the push and pull patterns creates a posture called upper cross syndrome.

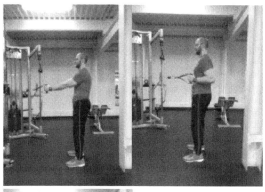

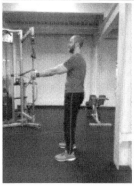

Core (anti-rotation and rotation)

The core consists of two movements – anti-rotation and rotation. Maintaining your postural stability and strength to prevent rotation is the definition of anti-rotation. It is important to be strong in this pattern prior to adding rotational movements in order to avoid potential damage to the spine.

The classic example for an anti-rotational exercise is the plank, which is pictured below. A rotational exercise is the exact opposite, meaning you employ an angular force with your body to create movement.

The classic example of rotational vs. anti-rotational is the golf swing. A golf swing is a rotational exercise, but in order to accomplish a safe and effective swing, you need to maintain postural stability, allowing the hips and shoulders to rotate around the body. That means the swing is an anti-rotational movement. If you don't possess postural stability through the golf swing, there is a greater chance of injury on the backswing and downswing, not to mention making it unlikely you'll break 100. Fore!

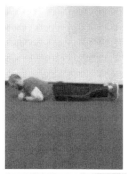
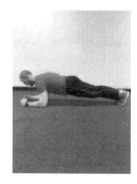
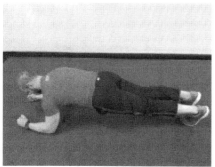

The Question: Machines or Bodyweight Exercises?

This is a question I get from nearly every client I train. Strength training machines require a controlled movement, and everything – the amount of resistance, seat height and range of motion – can be adjusted to the user's comfort. Talk about comfort, some machines even have a cup holder!

Machines can be a good starting point in helping you establish a strength training routine, and they're great if you're a beginner and don't have access to a personal trainer. But be sure to work with someone who can explain how the machines work and recommend the settings you should use. Make some notes you can refer to until you get the hang of the whole thing.

Bodyweight exercises are ideal when beginning a program, because your body is the ultimate gym. Bodyweight exercises are simply those that use your weight to provide resistance against gravity. I like bodyweight exercises because your body is the best strength training resistance and machine.

Do consult a personal trainer before beginning a bodyweight routine, and don't undertake one if you don't have pain-free range of motion. You can always add bodyweight training as you get stronger. Classic bodyweight exercises are the squat, hip hinge, push-up, pull-up and the plank.

Fit Tip

Strength training can be performed using machines, cables, bands, free weights and even body weight. There is not one training machine or apparatus that trumps all others; each piece has its pros and cons. The best methodology to strength training is to mix it up and add variety. Remember, it's the body's job to adapt to the exercise induced stress and stimulus, and it's your job to continually change the exercise induced stress and stimulus.

Let's Talk About Cardiovascular Exercise

Cardiovascular exercise is essential to your heart and pulmonary health and well-being. The American College of Sports Medicine recommends that everyone participate in at least 30 minutes a day of walking. However, if that seems daunting to start, scale it back. You can start with just 10-15 minutes of walking or low impact cardio.

Low impact cardio includes the elliptical machine, stationary bike or even the rowing machine. Walking should also be incorporated into active daily living. If there are orthopedic limitations, low impact cardio is an excellent alternative. There is less force and pounding on the joints, making it much easier to complete the exercise.

Exercise Intensity

Now that we've established some basics to get you moving, let's have a look at exercise intensity. If your doctor has cleared you to start an exercise program and you're a beginner, you'll want to keep your exercise intensity in the low to moderate range. To understand what that means, you need to know your age-predicted heart rate maximum, or maximum heart rate.

Figuring out your maximum heart rate isn't an exact science. The formula you use to come up with a ballpark number of your maximum heart rate is to subtract your age from 220. A 65-year-old, for instance, would have a maximum heart rate of about 155 beats per minute

Once you've figured out your maximum heart rate, you can use an activity tracker that includes a heart rate monitor to gauge the intensity at which you're exercising. If you're exercising on a treadmill, stationary bike or elliptical machine, the machine may include a heart rate monitor. Or, you can gauge your exercise intensity by paying attention to how you feel.

Check This Out

There is an inverse relationship between exercise intensity and duration: The higher the intensity, the shorter the duration of the workout. When starting an exercise routine, focus primarily on duration (i.e. number of minutes of cardio) and frequency (i.e. how many days of the week you exercise). Ideally, you want to be able to perform 30 minutes of cardio comfortably, for 4-5 days a week before raising the intensity of your workout. Barring medical limitation, increasing exercise intensity is beneficial to burning more calories, boosting metabolism and improving cardiovascular health.

So, calculate your maximum heart rate, and then check out the equations below to get an idea of the intensity at which you should be exercising.

Light intensity is a heart rate that is 57 - <64% of your heart rate max.

Moderate intensity is a heart rate that is 64 - <76% of your heart rate max.

Vigorous intensity is a heart rate that is 76 - <96% of your heart rate max.

Sample Calculation:

age: 65

220 - 65 = 155 HR max

Light Intensity: 88-99 bpm

155 beats per minute x .57 = 88

155 bpm x .64 = 99

Moderate Intensity:99-117 bpm

155 bpm x .64 = 99

155 bpm x .76 = 117

Vigorous Intensity: 117-148 bpm

155 bpm x .76 = 117

155 bpm x .96 = 148

Heart Rate Table				
Age	60% Light Intensity	70% Moderate Intensity	80% Vigorous Intensity (challenging)	90% Vigorous Intensity (very difficult)
50	102	119	136	153
55	99	116	132	149
60	96	112	128	144

65	93	109	124	140
70	90	105	120	135
75	87	102	116	131

Putting it all Together

If you're feeling a little confused right about now, don't worry. We've covered a lot of material. Let's recap the highlights of this chapter.

When incorporating an exercise

program into your weekly routine, keep it simple.

You don't need to complete every exercise every time you're at the gym.

If you plan to go to the gym three times per week, complete three exercises at each visit.

To start, do 2-3 sets of 10 repetitions of each of the three exercises, and 15-20 minutes of cardiovascular exercise.

Stick to that routine for one to two weeks, and then add one more exercise, increasing from three to four with the same number of sets and repetitions.

Add five to 10 minutes to your cardiovascular exercise after the first week.

Doing this provides a methodical, consistent and low-barrier approach to get you started. Remember that the key is establishing a routine. You can always add more to the program later. Below are two sample beginner workouts to try. The format consists of a warmup, balance exercise, two strength exercises, and then a cool down. As the program becomes easy and you're feeling confident, add an additional strength exercise. The goal is to build your strength routine to eight to 10 exercises, and one to two balance exercises.

Remember the 21-90 Rule

You don't have to complete every exercise and workout every day. Utilize the 21-90 rule to get started and keep going. It takes 21 days to build a habit and 90 days to turn it into a lifestyle. Going to the gym seven days a week will not, in most cases, build a habit, but it will burn you out. Ask yourself, how much can you do that's manageable when it comes to exercising.

That might mean exercising for 10 minutes a day for two to three days per week, or completing 150 minutes of cardio per week and strength training for three to four times per week.

Start with what you can do, and more importantly, what you enjoy and tolerate. This builds the habit and you can always add more time to your workouts or another day in your routine later. Maintaining your newly formed routine for 90 days will assure it becomes a part of your lifestyle. This is key. If it's part of your lifestyle, then it's a priority, and it will be easier to be consistent in exercising!

Day 1: Beginner

Warmup: Elliptical, 10-15 minutes

Your warmup is designed to increase your core temperature, your plasticity and your pliability. Low impact cardio is beneficial for the warmup because you're not placing unnecessary impact force on the joints. The warmup should start at low intensity and progress to moderate intensity.

Single leg balance: 3 x 20-30 seconds

Standing on one leg, lift the opposite knee to hip height. If you have difficultly lifting your knee to hip height, don't fret. Just lift the opposite foot off the ground so it is hovering above the floor.

Squats: 2-3 x 10 reps

Don't worry about depth or resistance, focus on pain-free range of motion.

Seated rows (machine): 2-3 x 10 reps

Cool down: Stationary bike, 10 minutes

This is often a neglected part of an exercise routine. Cooling down allows your mind and body to transition from an elevated, high intense state to your normal day-to-day baseline. Intensity should be from moderate to low intensity.

Day 2: Beginner

Warmup: Elliptical, 10-15 minutes

Balance quarter squat with eyes closed: 3 x 20 reps

This balance exercise challenges our propriocep-tive balance (how your brain and body determine where you are in space). Proprioception balance is usually the first aspect of balance to degrade as we age, because we rely on our eyes to assess where we are in our environment.

Split squats: 2-3 x 10 reps

Don't worry about depth or resistance, instead pain-free range of motion.

Chest press (machine): 2-3 x 10 reps

Cool down: Stationary bike, 10 minutes

Below is a sample exercise program, designed to be used at a gym. This program is advanced compared to the recommendations from above. Remember, less is more. Complete what you feel is comfortable within your abilities. You can always ADD more ex-ercises, reps, sets and intensity. There are two work-outs below. Start off with two days a week (Day 1 and Day 2). Complete two consistent weeks with the same routine. On the third week, add a third day of strength training; either day one or day two.

Day 1: Moderate to Advanced Programming

Warmup: Elliptical, 10-15 minutes

Single leg balance: 3 x 20-30 seconds

Squats: 2-3 x 10 reps

Seated rows (machine): 2-3 x 10 reps

Chest press (machine): 2-3 x 10 reps

Walking lunges: 2 x 10 reps

Lat pulldown (machine): 2 x 10 reps

Plank: 3 x 20 reps

This exercise provides core anti-rotation

Cool down: Stationary bike, 10 minutes

Day 2: Moderate to Advanced Programming

Warmup: Elliptical, 10-15 minutes

Balance quarter squat with eyes closed: 3 x 20 reps

Single arm deadlift: 2-3 x 10 reps

The deadlift exercise is a hip hinge pattern. Don't worry about heavy weight when learning this exercise, just focus on pain-free range of motion and securing your posture. Don't worry about depth or resistance, ether. Again, focus instead on pain-free range of motion.

Split squats: 2-3 x 10 reps

Standing rows (machine): 2-3 x 10 reps

Chest press (machine): 2-3 x 10 reps

Side planks: 2-3 x 20 reps

This exercise can be completed on the forearm or hand. Make sure hips and shoulders are perpendicular to the floor. This exercise provides core anti-rotation

Bird dogs: 3 x 10 reps

This exercise provides core anti-rotation

Cool down: Stationary Bike, 10 minutes

Wrapping it Up

I hope that this chapter has given you an understanding of how to calculate an age-predicted heart rate max, along with providing some basic balance and strength exercises and explaining how to design a program to start your routine.

It's a lot of information, but I hope you see that if you take it one exercise or one routine at a time, the material will seem simpler and more manageable.

In our final chapter, we'll discuss gym 101, which is what you should expect when entering a health/fitness club for the first time. You'll also learn about choosing a gym and how to find a personal trainer who can make sure you get – and stay – on the right track.

Let's finish strong!

CHAPTER 8:
CHOOSING A GYM
AND FINDING A
TRAINER

"The reason I exercise is for the quality of life I enjoy."

- Kenneth H. Cooper, physician and author of "Aerobics"

So, you're ready to commit to an exercise program. Congratulations! Your body, mind and emotional health will thank you for it.

To find a gym that will be a good fit, I strongly recommend researching the clubs in your area before committing to one. Read consumer reviews, visit the company's website and, if you know others who belong to a particular gym, pick their brains. What do they like about it? Are staff members willing to help? Is it clean? When does it get the most crowded?

Why the extensive research? Because when attempting to make a lifestyle change, it's best to have the optimal conditions to help assure you'll be successful. For example, if you're quiet and low key, the last place you'll want to work out is a stereotypical meathead gym with loud music and usually poor decisions. If the gym is too far from your home, that could be an excuse for you to slack off.

The maintenance of a club and the helpfulness and demeanor of its staff are usually indicative of how a gym is performing.

If the facility is dirty and unkempt, morale among staff and patrons is likely to be low. Apathy regarding the cleanliness of a gym isn't good, as it can indicate issues regarding the sanitary conditions of equipment.

Staff is a huge factor in terms of your comfort level

John Monteleone

about joining, showing up and remaining a member of a particular gym. If there is high turnover of staff, the quality of service is likely to decline. Trust your gut. You can pick up the vibe of a facility by the staff at the front door. If the employees are friendly, warm and personable, there's a good chance that gym might be the place for you.

On the other hand, if the folks at the front desk are buried in their phones, lack social skills or are flat-out rude, you'd be better off to look for another workout facility.

Equipment also is key to a successful gym. If exercise equipment is consistently broken and not repaired in a timely manner, that's a concern.

Again, pay attention to cleanliness. Remember that a lot of people touch the machines with sweaty hands and other body parts; sanitizing wipes should be readily available so clients can clean a machine after using it.

Be sure there is someone available to give you a tutorial on the equipment so you can avoid injury and get the most effective workout possible. Hospitality is key for a gym and necessary in order for you to feel comfortable and welcomed.

GYM 101

So, what should you expect when you first set foot into a gym? Keep in mind that all gyms are not the same. There are clubs that are dirty and dingy, while others are clean, pristine and well lighted.

Here are some things to look for when deciding on a gym.

The Basics

Most gyms provide a locker room where you can shower and change, and lockers to secure your belongings while exercising.

When it comes to cardio equipment, most gyms provide treadmills, ellipticals, stationary bikes and recumbent bikes.

Strength training equipment normally includes a pin-loaded circuit, cable machines, dumbbells, kettlebells and plate-loaded equipment. There should be a variety of equipment to break up monotony

Most gyms provide access to Wi-Fi for your mobile devices, which will allow you to listen to music or watch your favorite TV shows and movies while getting your cardio workout in. The Wi-Fi password for gym members is usually listed at the front desk, and staff should give you a hand if you have trouble logging onto the network.

Using the Equipment

It's important not to "hog up" the equipment. For example, if you're using a piece of exercise equipment, you don't have to rush through your workout, but don't dawdle, either.

And when you're finished, please don't slam the weights or machines. The cacophony promotes a less-than-ideal gym environment, and it also can damage the equipment.

Making sure you clean the equipment is super important to gym etiquette. Health clubs operating at an elite level provide in-house cleaning to make sure the gym remains immaculate.

But members should still clean their equipment after using it. It's highly recommended from a hygiene and germ safety perspective, but it's also a courtesy toward fellow members. This simple act reinforces a positive culture within the health club and maintains the equipment that aids in improving your health.

Fashion Statement

What you wear doesn't have to be spandex, tight shorts and tight tops. Gym clothing is casual and relaxed, which I define as shorts, T-shirts, sneakers and perhaps a towel for perspiration.

You don't have to be scantily clad to work out. I think gym attire should reflect a blue collar mindset. Wear something that makes you feel ready to work and sweat.

That said, there's nothing wrong with being stylish at a gym, as long as your outfit is functional.

Cellphones

They could be a necessity if you want to listen to music or stream a movie while working out. However, if you need to talk on the phone, go outside the gym or in the locker room.

Thought for the Day

Based on my career experience and personal preferences, I am biased toward small-business gyms, compared to big box corporate gyms. That doesn't mean a big box gym isn't capable of providing a great service, but in my opinion, if you want a more personal experience and a real sense of belonging, support the local gym. Local health clubs tend to have members that encompass the community and provide familiarity; so choose the place that makes you feel the most comfortable and secure.

Pay attention to the type of equipment a club has available. If the gym is mostly pull-up bars, squat racks, medicine balls and hammer strength equipment, that may not be the best place for you. Ideally, the gym you choose will have a variety of equipment to meet the needs of all its clients.

Squat racks are great, but there also should be pin-loading machines, a stretching area, treadmills, recumbent bikes and elliptical machines.

The functionality of the equipment is key, as well. Is the equipment easy to use? Can you understand how to use it? If you're using a leg press, for instance, your legs should bear the brunt of the resistance, not your chest.

What to Look for When Choosing a Personal Trainer

OK. I've been waiting for eight chapters to write about choosing a personal trainer, because it's a topic I feel strongly about.

Remember that no two trainers are created equal, and there are multiple factors to consider when choosing one. Just like an iceberg, there's more to a personal trainer than is visible from the surface; selecting yours should be a rigorous process.

I think it's that important because, literally, your fitness professional will have your health in his or her hands. You'll want to meet prospective trainers and spend a little time with each one before making a decision. Get a feel for the trainer and decide if you feel comfortable.

Don't ever let a gym manager or other staff member pair you with a personal trainer who you've never met or spent some time with just because that trainer is available to take new clients. Essentially, when you agree to work with a personal trainer, you are hiring someone who will be working for you. An interview prior to making the hire is essential.

Let's look at some of the things you should consider before agreeing to work with a personal trainer:

Personality

If you interview a trainer who has the personality of mud, you should definitely keep looking. Personality can be just as important as credentials and training experience. If you and the trainer don't communicate well, how can you expect to reach your health and fitness goals?

Especially in the beginning, you need someone who can motivate you and keep you involved and enthusiastic.

Your trainer should be sociable and extroverted, with an easy ability to engage in conversation. The trainer should show a keen interest in you, your health and your fitness goals.

Empathy is another important character trait. If you're just starting to exercise and don't feel comfortable, a trainer should be aware and sensitive to your situation. Your care and the realization of your goals should be your primary focus as a client.

If your trainer isn't on board with those things or doesn't seem genuinely concerned about your personal well-being, it's time to look for a different trainer.

Education and Experience

Education and experience set one trainer apart from another. If you're going to commit to a trainer, be sure you find a professional and not someone who moonlights or dabbles in the trade. A professional is a personal trainer who eats, sleeps and breathes training and other aspects of the fitness industry.

An individual who does training on the side while spending most of his/her time doing something else isn't able to commit the energy and focus necessary for you to succeed.

It's unlikely that you'd choose a doctor who practices medicine on the side, and it's the same with a personal trainer.

Working with a professional gives you confidence and loyalty, along with the knowledge that you'll accomplish your goals safely and efficiently.

Credentials and Certifications

There is a significant difference between a trainer who has credentials and one who has a certificate. Certifications are obtained when a trainer purchases a program in the form of a one- or two-day seminar. By simply purchasing the seminar and attending, a certificate is awarded.

To earn a credential, on the other hand, the trainer studies for three to six months prior to an examination. The exam is difficult and typically results in a low pass rate. Trainers who do pass have demonstrated competency in a specialized discipline within the health and fitness industry.

A credentialed personal trainer is someone who clearly went the extra mile and did the hard work of earning that status, demonstrating a commitment to the profession.

Once a trainer has become credentialed, he/she is obligated to earn certifications for continuing education. In that case, certifications make sense, as those courses broaden the trainer's knowledge and practice.

Certifications, however, shouldn't be the only education a personal trainer receives. Just as attending a seminar on basic home repair doesn't make you a contractor, attending a course on fitness training doesn't make someone a personal trainer. Look for credentials, the gold standard of personal training.

Fitness Degrees

The health and fitness industry has evolved to the point where many colleges and universities offer degree programs for students who want to become personal trainers.

It may seem hard to comprehend, but yes, many personal trainers have earned undergraduate, and in some cases, master's degrees in a field related to health and fitness. Some of those degrees are kinesiology (my field of study and degree), exercise science, biomechanics, health and wellness, exercise psychology and exercise physiology.

Obviously, I recommend seeking a trainer who has obtained an undergraduate or master's degree in the health and fitness industry.

More about Credentials

There are several organizations that award reputable credentials. The National Strength and Conditioning Association (NSCA), American College of Sports Medicine (ACSM), National Academy of Sports Medicine (NASM) and the American Council on Exercise (ACE) are my personal recommendations for organizations that provide reputable credentials.

Credentials are similar to health and fitness degrees, regarding unique perspective and specialty knowledge and experience.

I have been a health and fitness professional for more than 10 years, but I have a bias like everyone else. The big three credentials I think a health and fitness professional should have are a Certified Strength and Conditioning Specialist credential from NSCA, a Certified Special Population Specialist credential from NSCA and an Exercise Physiologist Certified credential from ACSM.

In my opinion, the Exercise Physiologist Certified credential is the gold standard. Why? The exercise prescription recommended for everyone is based off some rigorous and strict research, and the ACSM guidelines started with specific populations, specifically cardiovascular patients.

Their scope of recommendations originally ranged from special populations and then moved to general populations. To clarify, special populations are individuals who are diagnosed with orthopedic or medical limitations such as hypertension, asthma or knee replacement.

Questions to Ask Before Hiring a Trainer

When you meet with a prospective trainer, be prepared with some questions. Here are some to consider:

How long have you worked as a personal trainer?

How many clients do you have?

Why did you want to become a personal trainer?

Do you have a health- and fitness-related degree?

What credentials do you have?

How do you motivate your clients to exceed their goals?

What's your personal philosophy regarding health and wellness?

Meet My Client: Mr. Smith

My 80-year old client, Mr. Smith retired from a career in sales and now spends his time volunteering on the grounds of the local museum. Every year he helps to transplant hundreds of plants from the greenhouse where they were started onto the museum grounds. A self-described "gym rat," he also spends a lot of time at the fitness center.

Mr. Smith has a favorite saying that he used to recite to encourage his co-workers: "Every day you have to slay the dragon." Instead of using that phrase now to apply to sales quotas, it's become his mantra regarding his exercise routine. And every day he shows up at the gym and does just that, enabling him to enjoy his life without limitations.

Gym Membership

OK, this is the part of the book where we dive into the business side of this industry. Brace yourself. Gym memberships come in all shapes and sizes.

I can't go into too much detail regarding the best memberships. However, I can provide some tips when joining a gym.

Always think money and time. If you're looking at a gym based off a price point, the longer your membership, the cheaper per month. The exact inverse is true if you're joining for an abbreviated time.

Most gym memberships can range from month to month, three months, six months or one-year commitments. What you pay for a membership varies greatly, depending on location, the type of facility and other factors. Gym memberships can range from $10 to hundreds of dollars a month.

Personally, I prefer a month-to-month membership because it puts the responsibility and accountability on the business to maintain consistent service and cleanliness. If the gym doesn't uphold its end of the agreement, then I know I can leave the following month.

But with three-month, six-month and one-year contracts, you're locked in until the term ends or you buy out your contract for a ridiculous amount of money.

Personal Training Fees

Personal training services are an additional service at a gym. Training memberships or fees can be based per session, number of sessions, per month or even a year contract.

I prefer the training services be per session. Again, let's place the accountability and responsibility on the professional to provide your specific care.

Training session rates can vary depending on geographical location. Rates in San Francisco will be higher than those in Reading, Pennsylvania.

Remember, you get what you pay for regarding service. For example, if the personal trainer possesses advanced credentials and expertise in a field, expect to pay more for the professional's guidance and service.

A Sunday Conversation with My Dad – Two Years Later

I was getting ready to head out for my Sunday morning walk when the phone rang. It was 5:30 a.m. Yep, it was my dad, and yeah, I know we're a strange breed.

It's autumn, and the air is crisp with a chill. The leaves are red, orange and yellow. My dad is now 62 years old, and he asks my advice about changing his lifestyle to be healthier and to maintain, or possibly increase, his energy throughout the day.

"You're a farmer and gunsmith," I remind him. "That's about as physically active as one can be at your age."

He shrugs off the comment.

We discuss the value of him adding apple cider vinegar to his diet, significantly reducing carbohydrate intake, making dinner the smallest meal and continuing to walk and move throughout the day.

The apple cider vinegar recommendation isn't met with any enthusiasm, so I explained the benefit of a natural probiotic and good gut health that results from consuming it.

"I tried it, son, it's not my cup of tea," he says.

To which I replied, "That's great! It's not supposed

John Monteleone

to taste like tea, Dad."

Sarcasm is spoken fluently in my family.

My dad is not only a farmer and a gunsmith, he recently decided to raise beef cattle. Yes, beef cattle. I am impressed with that.

Not only did he reinvent himself and create a completely different career after retirement, he continues to evolve. I think that's an interesting perspective to this journey that demonstrates if you keep growing as an individual, you maintain your youth.

Remember that happiness is found in progressing – not in perfection. And, progress is found in keeping physically active. When we are constantly learning, moving and exercising, I think we find a special happiness.

"I have to keep moving son, gotta stay active," my father says, as he does during nearly every conversation we have.

And he's right. He does need to keep moving to stay active, because that's the silver lining in life, and especially in retirement. When you keep moving, you can keep up with life and all its joys and challenges. If you don't stay active, life will pass you by – mentally, physically and emotionally.

I'm still young – in my 30s -- but I've learned a lot from observing my dad and working with my older clients. They've taught me that life is to be enjoyed, and there are many, many ways to assure your life will be meaningful. To achieve that, however, you need to have the positive habits and lifestyle to support it.

At the end of the day, exercise is not a "coulda, shoulda, woulda" proposition; it's a must-do in order to stay active and involved.

It's never too late.

References

Chapter 1:

President's Council on Sports, Fitness & Nutrition
https://www.hhs.gov/fitness/resource-center/
facts-and-statistics/index.html

Medical News Today: Report on Prevalence of Type
2 Diabetes
Berry, Jennifer, April 1, 2019.

Sitting Time, Physical Activity, and Risk of Mortality in Adults
Emmanuel Stamatakis, Joanne Gale, Adrian
Bauman, Ulf Ekelund, Mark Hamer and Ding Ding
http://www.onlinejacc.org/content/73/16/2062

Physical Inactivity: Associated Diseases and Disorders
Knight, Joseph A.
http://www.annclinlabsci.org/
content/42/3/320.full

CDC report on the prevalence of prediabetics https://www.cdc.gov/diabetes/data/statistics-report/prevalence.html

Chapter 2:

The History of Fitness

Dalleck, Lance C. M.S. and Kravitz, Len Ph.D.

Chapter 3:

Sedentary Behavior: Emerging Evidence for a New Health Risk
Owen, Neville PhD, Sparling, Phillip B. EdD, Healy, Geneve N. PhD, Dunstan, David W. PhD. and Charles E. Matthews, PhD
https://www.ncbi.nlm.nih.gov/pmc/articles/PMC2996155/

The History of Fitness
Dalleck, Lance C. M.S. and Kravitz, Len Ph.D.

New Survey: To Sit or Stand? Almost 70% of Full Time American Workers Hate Sitting, but They do it all Day Every Day

Simple Changes Can Make a Big Difference in Health and Productivity
https://www.prnewswire.com/news-releases/new-survey-to-sit-or-stand-almost-70-of-full-time-american-workers-hate-sitting-but-they-do-it-all-day-every-day-215804771.html
St. Paul, MN., July 17, 2013, PRNewswire

Lower Cross and Upper Cross Syndrome
Janda Syndromes
http://www.jandaapproach.com/the-janda-

approach/jandas-syndromes/

2019 Physical Activity Council's Overview Report on U.S. Participation
The Physical Activity Council's annual study tracking sports, fitness, and recreation participation in the U.S.
http://www.physicalactivitycouncil.com/pdfs/current.pdf

CBS News, May 3, 2013
Jaslow, Ryan
https://www.cbsnews.com/news/cdc-80-percent-of-american-adults-dont-get-recommended-exercise/

Chapter 5:

ACSM Guidelines for Exercise Testing and Prescription 9th ed
 LWW; Ninth edition, February 9, 2013, Philadelphia, PA

Physical Activity Instruction of Older Adults
Human Kinetics, Champaign, IL, 2005
Jones, Jessie C, Rose, Debra J.

Chapter 7:

ACSM Guidelines for Exercise Testing and Prescription 9th ed

LWW; Ninth edition, February 9, 2013, Philadelphia, PA